The Clean Eating Cookbook & Diet

Over 60 Healthy Whole Food Recipes

✦ antarespress

Copyright © 2014 by Antares Press.

All rights reserved.

No part of this publication may be reproduced, stored in a retrieval system or transmitted in any form or by any means, electronic, mechanical, photocopying, recording, scanning or otherwise, except as permitted under Sections 107 or 108 of the 1976 United States Copyright Act, without the prior written permission of the Publisher.

Limit of Liability/Disclaimer of Warranty: The Publisher and the author make no representations or warranties with respect to the accuracy or completeness of the contents of this work and specifically disclaim all warranties, including without limitation warranties of fitness for a particular purpose. No warranty may be created or extended by sales or promotional materials. The advice and strategies contained herein may not be suitable for every situation. This work is sold with the understanding that the publisher is not engaged in rendering medical, legal or other professional advice or services. If professional assistance is required, the services of a competent professional person should be sought. Neither the Publisher nor the author shall be liable for damages arising herefrom. The fact that an individual, organization or website is referred to in this work as a citation and/or potential source of further information does not mean that the author or the Publisher endorses the information the individual, organization or website may provide or recommendations they/it may make. Further, readers should be aware that Internet websites listed in this work may have changed or disappeared between when this work was written and when it is read.

Antares Press publishes its books in a variety of electronic and print formats. Some content that appears in print may not be available in electronic books, and vice versa.

TRADEMARKS: Antares Press and the Antares Press logo are trademarks or registered trademarks in the United States and other countries, and may not be used without written permission. All other trademarks are the property of their respective owners. Antares Press is not associated with any product or vendor mentioned in this book.

CONTENTS

Introduction 11

Chapter 1: Breakfasts

Zucchini & Apple Pancakes with Turkey Bacon 16

Shrimp & Artichoke Quesadillas 18

Clean Breakfast Burrito 20

Honey Almond Cornmeal Porridge 22

Carrot Date Breakfast Bars 23

Grains and Berries Cereal Blend 24

Clean Omelet 25

Chapter 2: Snacks

Clean Style Corn Bread 30

Black-Eyed Peas Salsa 32

No-Bake Power Balls 33

Mango Pineapple Ice Pops 34

Hummus and Cucumber Bruschetta 35

Flaxseed Crackers 37

Cantaloupe Ice Cream 38

Coco-Papaya Pudding 39

Chapter 3: Salads

Escarole Salad 42

Grilled Tuna with Chickpea and Spinach Salad 43

Caribbean-Style Tabbouleh 45

Moroccan Lentil Salad 47

Asparagus and Orange Salad With Ginger 48

Quick Shrimp Ceviche Stuffed Avocados........................... 50

Mango Avocado Salad 52

Apple Cucumber Salad 53

Cucumber Quinoa Salad 54

Chapter 4: Soups and Stews

Carrot and Dill Soup 58

Spinach and Dulse Soup... 59

Seafood and Black Bean Chili.. 60

Tokyo Beef and Noodle Soup 62

Spiced Pork Stew.. 64

Moroccan Chicken Stew with Couscous 66

Chicken Soup 68

Quick Cold Green Soup 69

Chapter 5: Main Dishes

Sesame Maple Salmon with Spinach.............................. 72

Braised Cod With Leeks.. 74

Clean Chicken in a Pot... 76

Grilled Chicken Breasts with Garlic 77

Grilled Scallops with Sauteed Asparagus & Peppers.... 78

Thyme Roasted Turkey Breasts 80

Marinated Flank Steak 81

Lettuce-Wrapped Beef and Pepper Fajitas 82

Pork Medallions and Peppers 84

Leg of Lamb 86

Grilled Lamb Chops 87

Chapter 6: Vegetables

Brussels Sprouts with Lemon 90

Veggie Medley 91

Sauteed Spinach 92

Parmesan Asparagus 93

Balsamic Rosemary Beets 94

Baked Tomatoes Gratin 95

Chapter 7: Desserts

Melon Cooler 98

Grilled Pineapple with Cinnamon Yogurt Sauce 99

Cherry Berry 100

Strawberry Peach Parfaits 101

Banana Coconut Ice Cream 102

Pumpkin Pie Puddings 103

Chapter 8: Smoothies

Clean Breeze Smoothie 106

Nutty Berry Smoothie 107

Mango-Kale Starter 108

Banana Spice Smoothie 109

Pear Green Tea Smoothie 110

Green Apple Smoothie 111

Ginger Pineapple Green 112

Green Smoothie 113

Standard U.S. / Metric Measurement Conversions............ 114

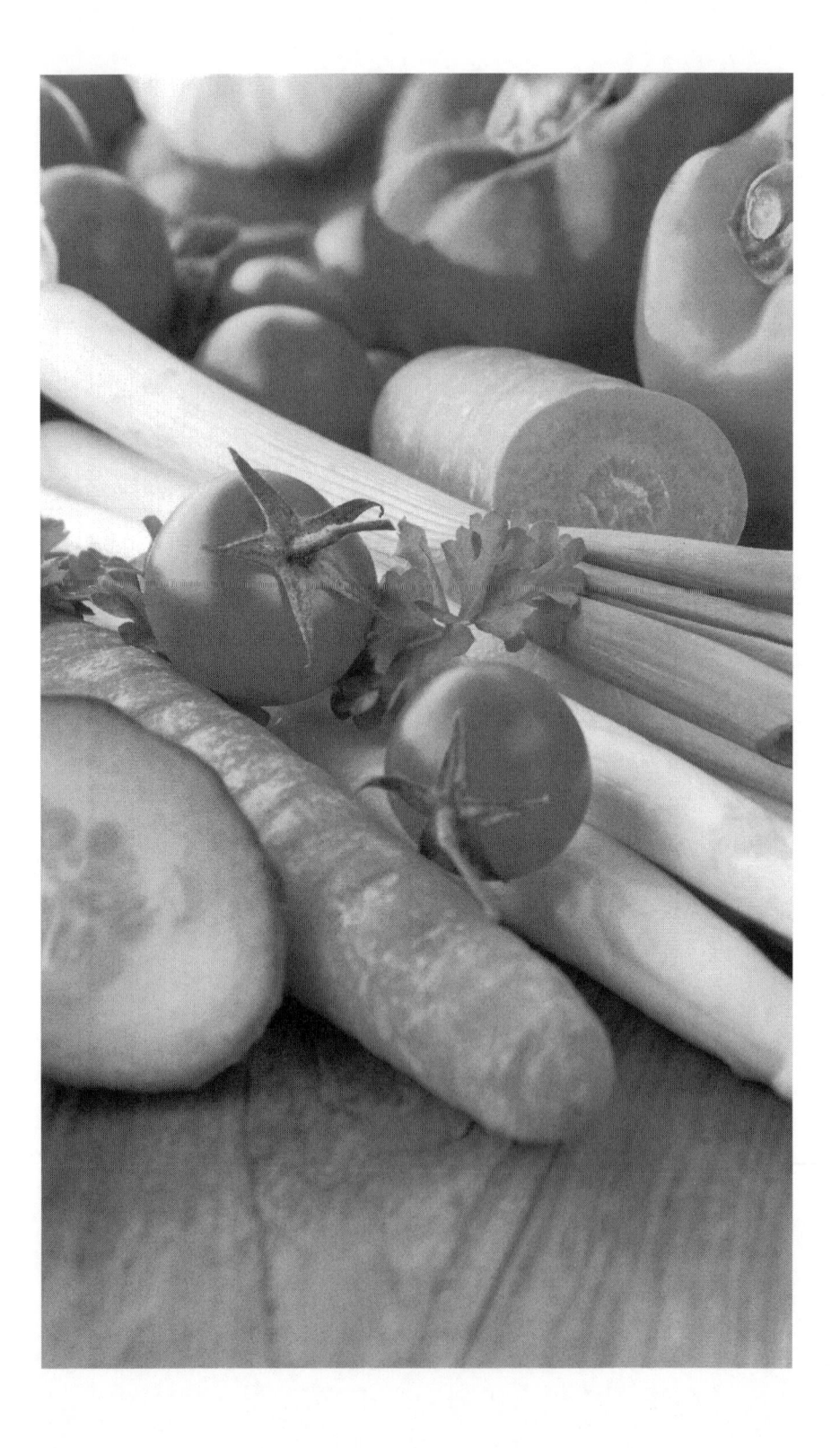

INTRODUCTION

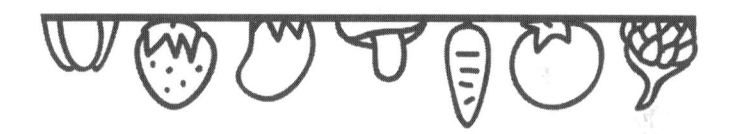

Fundamentals of Clean Eating

INTRODUCTION

FUNDAMENTALS OF CLEAN EATING!

Clean eating might be the best solution if you're ready for a lifestyle change that will help you get in the healthiest condition of your life.

If you choose this lifestyle you'll eat great tasting meals without feeling hungry or deprived. You'll enjoy the many benefits of caring for yourself with nutritious whole food.

WHAT IS CLEAN EATING?

Clean Eating is a simple concept: eat whole, minimally processed foods that contains natural ingredients. This is good for you and for the planet. **Eat five to six times a day** – three meals and two to three small snacks. You should include in your meal a lean protein, enough fresh fruit and vegetables, and a complex carb to keep you energized all day long. There are 3 big rules for clean eating:

A) Foods closest to their natural state

The more processed foods are, the less naturally occurring vital nutrients and the more harmful ingredients they contain. The ingredients on the label should sound familiar. If you can't pronounce an ingredient it's a sign that you shouldn't eat it. Choose foods with ingredients you find in most home kitchens.

Ingredients to avoid:
» partially hydrogenated oil
» refined added sugars and salt
» artificial sweeteners (acesulfame K, saccharin, aspartame)
» artificial food coloring (Blue 2, Green 3, Red 3, Yellow 5 and 6)
» nitrates and nitrites in cured meats

B) Eat a rainbow: enjoy colorful foods

Eating a variety of colorful food provides a unique blend of vitamins, minerals, antioxidants and phytochemicals that will boost your immunity. Different colored foods play different roles in your body. Choose more natural colors for a more varied and inclusive diet.

C) Choose local and seasonal foods

Why to choose local and seasonal? Because most foods taste better and contain higher amounts of nutrients. They are fresh and leave a smaller carbon footprint (travel shorter distances). Choose foods from your country or even better from within your region (best within 30 miles radius).

CHAPTER 1

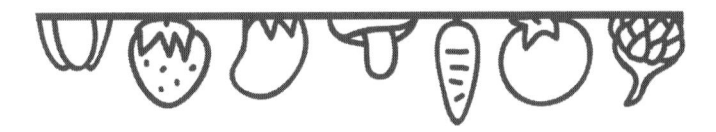

Breakfasts

ZUCCHINI & APPLE PANCAKES WITH TURKEY BACON

BREAKFASTS › TURKEY BACON, MAPLE SYRUP, CANE JUICE, NUTMEG, CINNAMON, EGG, MILK, ZUCCHINI, APPLE, RICOTTA

SERVES: 8

8 1-ounce strips turkey bacon

1 tablespoon maple syrup

olive oil cooking spray

1 1/2 cups light spelt flour

2 tablespoons baking powder

1 tablespoon organic evaporated cane juice

1/2 teaspoon ground nutmeg

1/2 teaspoon ground cinnamon

1/8 teaspoon sea salt

1 large egg

1 cup 1% milk

2 teaspoons safflower oil

1 cup coarsely grated zucchini

1 cup coarsely grated apple (Gala / Honeycrisp)

1/2 cup reduced-fat ricotta cheese

Preheat oven to 400 degrees F. On a parchment-lined baking sheet, arrange bacon spaced apart in a single layer. Bake, turning once, until just beginning to crisp, about 7 minutes. Remove from oven and brush with maple syrup. Continue baking to desired crispness. Cover to keep warm.

Meanwhile, mist a griddle with cooking spray and heat to medium-high.

In a medium bowl, sift together flour, baking powder, cane juice, nutmeg, cinnamon and salt. In a separate bowl, combine egg, milk and oil, whisking to combine. Mix wet ingredients into dry, whisking until just combined. Fold in zucchini, apple and ricotta.

Working in batches, drop 3 tablespoons batter per pancake on griddle. Cook until golden brown on bottom, then flip and continue cooking until golden brown on other side and cooked through, about 4 to 5 minutes total. Serve with bacon alongside.

Breakfasts

SHRIMP & ARTICHOKE QUESADILLAS

BREAKFASTS › CREAM CHEESE, GREEK YOGURT, GARLIC, LEMON JUICE, RED PEPPER FLAKES, SPINACH, SHRIMP, ARTICHOKES, MOZZARELLA, TORTILLAS

SERVES: 12

- 3 ounces low-fat cream cheese, softened
- 1/2 cup nonfat plain Greek yogurt
- 2 cloves garlic, minced
- 1 teaspoon fresh lemon juice
- 1/2 teaspoon red pepper flakes
- 5 ounces frozen chopped spinach, thawed and squeezed of excess liquid
- 4 oz cooked shrimp (peeled, deveined and tails removed), roughly chopped
- 4 1/2 ounces frozen artichokes, thawed and roughly chopped
- 1/4 cup shredded part-skim mozzarella cheese
- 12 6-inch corn tortillas
- 6 teaspoons olive oil, divided

Heat oven on lowest (warm) setting. To a medium bowl, add cream cheese and beat with an electric hand mixer on high for

1 minute until fluffy. Add yogurt and blend on high until smooth, about 1 more minute. Reduce mixer speed to medium and mix in garlic, lemon juice and pepper flakes. With a spatula, fold in spinach, shrimp, artichokes and mozzarella.

Place one tortilla on a work surface and brush with 1/2 teaspoon oil. Flip over so that oiled side is facing down. Spread 1/3-cup spinach-artichoke mixture evenly over tortilla. Top with second tortilla and brush top with 1/2 teaspoon oil. Repeat with remaining tortillas.

Heat a large (12-inch) cast iron skillet on medium. In batches, carefully transfer quesadillas to skillet. Cook for 4 to 6 minutes, turning once, until lightly browned. Transfer to a cutting board and cool for 1 minute. Cut each quesadilla into four pieces, and place on a baking sheet in oven to keep warm while cooking remaining quesadillas.

CLEAN BREAKFAST BURRITO

BREAKFASTS › TURKEY, CUMIN, GARLIC POWDER, BLACK PEPPER, BLACK BEANS, RED PEPPERS, SPINACH, HUMMUS, TORTILLA

SERVES: 4

olive oil cooking spray

6 ounces extra lean ground turkey

1 teaspoon ground cumin

1/4 teaspoon garlic powder

4 egg whites

1/4 teaspoon sea salt

1/8 teaspoon freshly ground black pepper

1/3 cup drained and rinsed black beans

1/3 cup drained and chopped roasted red peppers

2 cups lightly packed fresh spinach

1/4 cup hummus, homemade or store bought

2 whole grain sprouted tortillas (such as Ezekiel), warmed (optional)

Chipotle Mexican hot sauce, to taste (optional)

Heat a large nonstick skillet over medium-high heat, and if necessary spray with olive oil cooking spray. Add ground turkey, cumin and garlic powder, and use a wooden spatula to break the meat into small pieces. Cook until no longer pink, two minutes.

Add egg whites to same skillet, season mixture with salt and pepper, and stir until opaque, two minutes. Add black beans, roasted red peppers and spinach, and stir all ingredients together.

Spread hummus on warm tortillas, then top with turkey mixture and top with chipotle hot sauce, if desired. Roll up burritos and eat warm.

HONEY ALMOND CORNMEAL PORRIDGE

BREAKFASTS › MILK, CORNMEAL, ALMONDS, HONEY, NUTMEG

SERVES: 4

4 cups milk

1/2 teaspoon salt

1/2 cup cornmeal

1/2 cup slivered almonds

3 tablespoons liquid honey

pinch ground nutmeg

In saucepan, bring milk and salt to boil. Whisk in cornmeal, almonds, honey and nutmeg, reduce heat and simmer, whisking constantly, for 4 to 5 minutes or until desired thickness.

CARROT DATE BREAKFAST BARS

BREAKFASTS › CINNAMON, DATES, EGGS, BROWN SUGAR, CARROTS

SERVES: 12 BARS

3/4 cup each all-purpose flour and whole wheat flour

2 teaspoons baking powder

1 1/2 teaspoon cinnamon

1 teaspoon baking soda

1 cup chopped dates

2 eggs

1/2 cup packed brown sugar

1/2 cup vegetable oil

2 cups grated carrots

In large bowl, whisk all-purpose and whole wheat flours, baking powder, cinnamon and baking soda; stir in dates. In separate bowl, whisk together eggs, sugar and oil; stir in carrots. Pour over dry ingredients; stir just until moistened. Spread in greased 8-inch (2 L) square metal cake pan.

Bake in centre of 350 degrees F oven until cake tester inserted in centre comes out clean, 45 to 50 minutes. Let cool in pan on rack. Cut into bars. (Make-ahead: Wrap individually in plastic wrap; store for up to 2 days.)

GRAINS AND BERRIES CEREAL BLEND

BREAKFASTS › WHOLE BRAN CEREAL, GRANOLA, CRANBERRIES

SERVES: 28 (1-CUP SERVINGS)

- 8 cups whole bran cereal
- 6 cups low-fat granola
- 4 cups wheat and barley nugget cereal (such as Grape Nuts)
- 7 cups seven-grain-and-sesame medley cereal (such as Kashi)
- 2 cups dried cranberries and/or raisins

Combine cereals and cranberries. Cover; store up to 2 weeks. Or seal in freezer bags; freeze up to 3 months.

CLEAN OMELET

BREAKFASTS › EGG WHITES, BASIL, BLACK PEPPER, GARLIC, RED ONION, RED BELL PEPPER, CHERRY TOMATOES

SERVES: 4

- **1 teaspoon extra-virgin olive oil**
- **2 cups egg whites**
- **1 teaspoon chopped fresh basil**
- **1/4 teaspoon freshly ground black pepper**
- **1/2 teaspoon minced garlic**
- **1/2 cup chopped yellow bell pepper**
- **1/2 cup finely chopped red onion**
- **1 cup halved cherry tomatoes**

Preheat the oven to broil.

In a large ovenproof skillet over medium heat, heat the olive oil.

In a medium bowl, thoroughly combine the egg whites, basil, and black pepper. Set aside.

Add the garlic and bell pepper to the skillet and saute until tender and fragrant, about 2 minutes. Add the onions and tomatoes and saute for another minute.

Remove the skillet from the heat and pour in the egg whites. Put the skillet back on the heat and cover it. Cook the omelet for 10 to 12 minutes without stirring, until egg mixture is set.

Remove the skillet from the heat and put it under the broiler for about 60 seconds, until the top is lightly browned.

Cut the omelet into quarters and transfer the pieces to plates.

Breakfasts

CHAPTER 2

Snacks

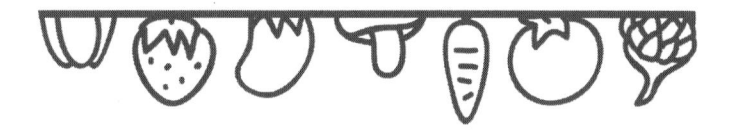

CLEAN STYLE CORN BREAD

SNACKS › ALMOND FLOUR, CORNMEAL, SEA SALT, EGGS, SOY MILK, MAPLE SYRUP, CANOLA OIL, JALAPENO PEPPER

SERVES: 16 (MAKES 16 PIECES)

extra-virgin olive oil for the baking dish

3/4 cup almond flour

1 1/4 cups cornmeal

1 tablespoon baking powder

pinch of sea salt

2 eggs

1 cup soy milk

3 tablespoons maple syrup

3 tablespoons canola oil

1/4 teaspoon chopped fresh jalapeno pepper

Preheat the oven to 425 degrees F.

Spread a thin coating of olive oil on the bottom and sides of an 8-inch-square baking dish.

In a large bowl, stir together the almond flour, cornmeal, baking powder, and salt. Make a well in the center of the dry ingredients and add the eggs, soy milk, maple syrup, canola oil, and jalapeno. Mix until the batter is well combined.

Spoon the batter into the baking dish. Bake the corn bread for 20 minutes.

Cut the corn bread into 2-inch squares and serve warm.

BLACK-EYED PEAS SALSA

SNACKS › BLACK-EYED PEAS, GREEN ONION, RED SWEET PEPPER, CIDER VINEGAR, JALAPENO, GARLIC, TORTILLA CRACKERS

SERVES: 16

1 15-ounce can black-eyed peas, rinsed and drained

1/4 cup thinly sliced green onions (2)

1/4 cup finely chopped red sweet pepper

2 tablespoons cooking oil

2 tablespoons cider vinegar

1 to 2 fresh jalapeños, seeded and chopped

1/4 teaspoon cracked black pepper

dash salt

2 cloves garlic, minced

Tortilla chips or assorted crackers

In a bowl combine black-eyed peas, green onions, sweet pepper, oil, vinegar, jalapeños, black pepper, salt, and garlic. Cover and chill overnight. Serve with tortilla chips.

NO-BAKE POWER BALLS

SNACKS › OATS, PUMPKIN SEEDS, CRANBERRIES, CURRANTS, FLAXSEED, NUT BUTTER, VANILLA

SERVES: 10

1/2 cup uncooked rolled oats

1/4 cup pumpkin seeds

1/4 cup dried unsweetened cranberries

1/4 cup dried unsweetened currants

1/4 cup organic hemp protein powder with fiber

1/4 cup millet

2 tablespoon roasted golden whole flaxseed

1/2 cup natural nut butter

1 tablespoon unsulfured blackstrap molasses

1/2 teaspoon real vanilla

Combine all dry ingredients in a medium-sized bowl, mixing well. Stir in nut butter, molasses and vanilla. Using your hands, knead mixture until well combined.

Using an ice cream scooper, portion out 10 equal-sized balls and place in an airtight container. Store in refrigerator or freezer. No need to thaw before eating.

MANGO PINEAPPLE ICE POPS

SNACKS › MANGO, PINEAPPLE JUICE, ORANGE JUICE, LIME JUICE

SERVES: 8 (MAKES 8 POPS)

2 pounds mango chunks

1 cup pineapple juice

1 cup freshly squeezed orange juice

1/4 cup freshly squeezed lime juice

Put all the ingredients in a blender and puree until smooth.

Pour the mixture into ice pop molds or plastic cups and freeze for 4 to 6 hours. Unmold the pops by briefly running warm water on the sides of the molds or cups. Eat immediately.

HUMMUS AND CUCUMBER BRUSCHETTA

SNACKS › FRENCH BAGUETTE, ITALIAN SEASONING, GARLIC POWDER, CUCUMBER, YOGURT, LEMON JUICE, OREGANO, HUMMUS

SERVES: 8

24 1/4-inch slices baguette French bread

olive oil nonstick cooking spray

1 tablespoon dried Italian seasoning, crushed

1/2 teaspoon garlic powder

2/3 cup finely chopped English cucumber

1/4 cup plain low-fat yogurt

1 tablespoon lemon juice

1 tablespoon snipped fresh oregano or 1 teaspoon dried oregano, crushed

3/4 cup quality hummus

snipped fresh oregano (optional)

Preheat oven to 400 degrees F. Arrange baguette slices in a single layer on a large baking sheet. Lightly coat slices with cooking spray. Combine Italian seasoning and garlic powder; sprinkle over bread slices. Bake about 10 minutes or until bread slices are crisp and light brown. Cool.

Meanwhile, in a small bowl combine cucumber, yogurt, lemon juice, and 1 tablespoon fresh oregano. Spread some of the hummus on top of each toasted baguette slice; top with cucumber mixture. If desired, sprinkle with additional oregano.

FLAXSEED CRACKERS

SNACKS › FLAXSEEDS, BUTTER, MILK

SERVES: 10 (MAKES ABOUT 40 PIECES)

1 1/2 cups all-purpose flour

1/4 cup flaxseeds

1/4 cup ground flaxseeds

4 teaspoons butter, softened

1/2 teaspoon baking powder

1/2 teaspoon salt

1/2 cup milk

¡In large bowl and using electric mixer, beat together flour, flax-seeds, ground flaxseeds, butter, baking powder and salt until crumbly. Add milk; mix until dough clumps together.

Turn out onto lightly floured surface; knead just until smooth. Wrap and refrigerate for 10 minutes.

Divide dough into quarters. On lightly floured surface, roll out dough, one-quarter at a time, to 1/8-inch (3 mm) thickness.

Transfer to ungreased rimless baking sheet. Bake in centre of 325 degrees F oven until golden and crisp, about 20 minutes.

Let cool on rack. Break into pieces.

CANTALOUPE ICE CREAM

SNACKS › COCONUT MILK, CANTALOUPE, HONEY

SERVES: 4

3 cups coconut or almond milk

1/2 cantaloupe, peeled, seeded, and diced

1/4 cup honey

Pulse all the ingredients in a food processor or blender until very smooth.

Pour the mixture into an ice cream maker and freeze according to the manufacturer's instructions.

Store the ice cream in an airtight container in the freezer until you're ready to eat it.

Scoop into bowls and serve.

COCO-PAPAYA PUDDING

SNACKS › COCONUT MILK, CANTALOUPE, HONEY

SERVES: 4

1 cup unsweetened almond milk

1 cup seeded, peeled, and diced fresh papaya

2 tablespoons chia seeds

2 tablespoons unsweetened shredded coconut

3 teaspoons honey

1/4 cup honey

In a medium bowl, mix together all the ingredients until well combined.

Cover the bowl and refrigerate for at least 6 hours, or overnight. Spoon the pudding into bowls and serve chilled.

CHAPTER 3

Salads

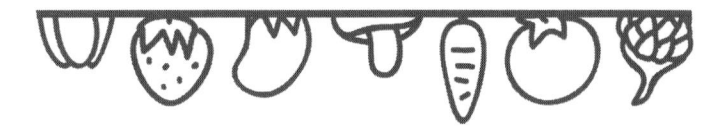

ESCAROLE SALAD

SALADS › GARLIC, ANCHOVY PASTE, HOT PEPPER SAUCE, ESCAROLE, ONION, RED/YELLOW PEPPER

SERVES: 2

2 tablespoons extra-virgin olive oil

4 teaspoons balsamic or wine vinegar

1 clove garlic, minced

1/4 teaspoon anchovy paste

dash hot pepper sauce

pinch each salt and pepper

half head escarole or romaine lettuce

quarter small sweet onion

half sweet red or yellow pepper

In large bowl, whisk together oil, vinegar, garlic, anchovy paste, hot pepper sauce, salt and pepper.

Cut escarole crosswise into thin strips. Thinly slice onion and red pepper. Add to bowl and mix well.

GRILLED TUNA WITH CHICKPEA AND SPINACH SALAD

SALADS › GARLIC, LEMON JUICE, OREGANO, TUNA STEAK, CHICKPEAS, SPINACH, TOMATO

SERVES: 4 (1 tuna steak, 1 cup salad per serving)

1 tablespoon olive or canola oil

1 tablespoon garlic, minced (about 2–3 cloves)

2 tablespoons lemon juice

1 tablespoon oregano, minced (or 1 tsp dried)

12 oz tuna steaks, cut into 4 portions (3 ounces each)

FOR SALAD:

1/2 can (15 1/2 ounces) low-sodium chickpeas (or garbanzo beans), drained and rinsed

1/2 bag (10 ounces) leaf spinach, rinsed and dried

1 tablespoon lemon juice

1 medium tomato, rinsed and cut into wedges

1/8 teaspoon salt

1/8 teaspoon ground black pepper

Preheat grill pan or oven broiler (with the rack 3 inches from heat source) on high temperature.

Combine oil, garlic, lemon juice, and oregano, and brush over tuna steaks. Marinate for 5–10 minutes.

Salads

Meanwhile, combine all salad ingredients. (Salad can be made up to 2 hours in advance and refrigerated.)

Grill or broil tuna on high heat for 3–4 minutes on each side until the flesh is opaque and separates easily with a fork (to a minimum internal temperature of 145 degrees F).

Serve one tuna steak over 1 cup of mixed salad.

CARIBBEAN-STYLE TABBOULEH

SALADS › BULGUR, MANGO, GREEN ONION, JALAPENO, ORANGE JUICE, TOMATO, CILANTRO, LETTUCE

SERVES: 6

3/4 cup bulgur

1 cup chopped, peeled mango

1/4 cup thinly sliced green onions

1/2 of a medium fresh jalapeño, seeded and finely chopped

2/3 cup orange juice

2 tablespoons canola oil or cooking oil

2 tablespoons lemon juice

1/4 teaspoon salt

1 medium tomato, seeded and chopped

1/4 cup snipped fresh cilantro

lettuce leaves (optional)

Place bulgur in a fine-mesh sieve or colander; rinse with cold water. Drain well. In a large bowl combine bulgur, mango, green onions, and jalapeño; set aside.

For dressing, in a screw-top jar combine orange juice, oil, lemon juice, and salt. Cover and shake well. Drizzle dressing over bulgur mixture; toss to coat. Cover and chill for 4 to 24 hours. Just before serving, gently stir tomato and cilantro into bulgur mixture. If desired, serve on lettuce-lined plates.

MOROCCAN LENTIL SALAD

SALADS › LENTILS, CHICKPEAS, RED&YELLOW BELL PEPPER, TOMATO, CUCUMBER, GREEN ONION, JALAPENO, LIME, CUMIN, CILANTRO

SERVES: 6

2 (15-ounce) cans sodium-free lentils, drained and rinsed

1 (15-ounce) can sodium-free chickpeas, drained and rinsed

1 red bell pepper, seeded and chopped

1 yellow bell pepper, seeded and chopped

2 tomatoes, seeded and chopped

1/2 cucumber, chopped

3 green onions, chopped

1 jalapeno pepper, minced

fresh juice of 2 limes

1 teaspoon ground cumin

1/2 teaspoon allspice

1/4 cup chopped fresh cilantro

Combine all the ingredients in a large bowl and stir to combine. Chill the salad for at least 30 minutes before serving.

ASPARAGUS AND ORANGE SALAD WITH GINGER

SALADS › ASPARAGUS, ORANGE, LETTUCE, AL-MONDS, GINGER, SOY SAUCE

SERVES: 6

1 1/2 pound asparagus

3 oranges

1 head Boston or Bibb lettuce

1/4 cup toasted sliced or slivered almonds

GINGER DRESSING:

2 tablespoons rice or cider vinegar

1 tablespoon grated ginger root

1/3 cup olive oil

1/2 teaspoon grated orange rind

2 teaspoons orange juice

1/2 teaspoon soy sauce

1/4 teaspoon each granulated sugar, salt and pepper

1/4 teaspoon hot pepper sauce

Snap off tough ends of asparagus; peel lower two-thirds of stems. In saucepan of boiling salted water, cook asparagus until tender-crisp, 2 to 3 minutes. Drain and chill under cold water; drain again and spread on towel to dry. (Make-ahead: Roll up in towel and refrigerate in plastic bag for up to 6 hours.)

GINGER DRESSING:

Mix vinegar with ginger; let stand for 2 minutes. Strain into bowl; press to extract liquid. Whisk in oil, rind and juice, soy sauce, sugar, salt, pepper and hot pepper sauce. (Make-ahead: Cover and refrigerate for up to 6 hours.)

Cut off peel and outside membrane of oranges; cut into 1/4-inch (5 mm) thick rounds. Place a few lettuce leaves on each plate; top with asparagus and oranges. Drizzle dressing over top. Sprinkle with almonds.

QUICK SHRIMP CEVICHE STUFFED AVOCADOS

SALADS › SHRIMP, RED PEPPER, RED&GREEN ONION, JALAPENO, TOMATO, CILANTRO, ORANGE&LIME JUICE, AVOCADO

SERVES: 4

- 1 pound jumbo cooked shrimp, peeled and deveined
- 1/2 red pepper, seeded and finely chopped
- 1/4 cup finely chopped red onion
- 1/4 cup finely chopped green onion
- 1/2 jalapeno pepper, seeded and finely chopped
- 1 tomato, finely chopped
- 2 tablespoons chopped cilantro
- juice of 1/2 orange (about 1/8 cup)
- juice of 2 limes (4 to 6 tablespoons)
- 1/2 teaspoon sea salt
- 1/4 teaspoon freshly ground black pepper
- 2 avocados

Remove shrimp tails and discard. Cut each shrimp into three or four pieces. In a bowl, combine shrimp with all other ingredients except avocados. Refrigerate for 15 minutes to allow flavors to combine.

Cut avocados in half and remove pits. Using a large spoon, scoop avocados out of their skins. Spoon ceviche into center of each avocado half, allowing it to overflow. Serve immediately..

MANGO AVOCADO SALAD

SALADS › MANGO, AVOCADO, LIME, CILANTRO, BLACK SESAME

SERVES: 2

2 ripe mangoes, peeled, pitted, and chopped

1 large avocado, peeled, pitted, and chopped

1 tablespoon lime juice

2 teaspoons olive oil

1 tablespoon cilantro leaves

1 tablespoon black sesame seeds

After you have the mangoes and avocado's chopped and pitted, simply mix all the ingredients together in a bowl and serve.

APPLE CUCUMBER SALAD

SALADS › APPLE, CUCUMBER, RED ONION, APPLE CIDER VINEGAR

SERVES: 1

1 apple, cored and diced

1 small cucumber, peeled and chopped with seeds removed

1/2 small red onion, diced

1 tablespoon apple cider vinegar

sea salt

In a bowl, toss all ingredients together and serve.

CUCUMBER QUINOA SALAD WITH OLIVES, FETA, MINT & OREGANO

SALADS › QUINOA, CUCUMBER, VEGETABLE BROTH, TOMATO, FETA CHEESE, KALAMATA OLIVES, MINT, OREGANO

SERVES: 10

1 cup dry quinoa, debris and discolored seeds removed

1 1/2 cups organic or reduced sodium vegetable broth

1 large cucumber, peeled, seeded, and chopped (1 1/2 cups)

1 large tomato, seeded and chopped (1 cup)

1/3 cup crumbled feta cheese

1/4 cup pitted Kalamata olives, sliced

2 tablespoons red wine vinegar

2 tablespoons extra-virgin olive oil

1 tablespoon chopped mint (or 1 teaspoon dried mint)

1/2 teaspoon salt

1/4 teaspoon dried oregano

Place quinoa in a medium saucepan, cover with water, and let soak for 5 minutes to prevent stickiness. Stir, then rinse in a colander with cool water, and drain. Return quinoa to the saucepan and add broth. Bring to a boil on high heat; reduce heat to low, cover, and cook for 20 minutes until quinoa is tender and liquid is completely absorbed. Spread quinoa on a plate to cool it quickly.

Place quinoa in a medium bowl and mix with the remaining ingredients. Chill for at least 30 minutes, up to 3 days.

CHAPTER 4

Soups and Stews

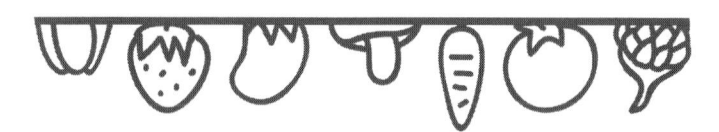

CARROT AND DILL SOUP

SOUPS AND STEWS › BUTTER, CELERY, ONION, GARLIC, CARROT, DILL, CHICKEN/ VEGGIE STOCK

SERVES: 8

2 tablespoons butter

3 stalks celery, chopped

2 onions, chopped

2 cloves garlic, minced

1/2 teaspoons each salt and pepper

5 cups chopped carrots (about 1 1/2 pound)

8 cups chicken or vegetable stock

1/4 cup chopped fresh dill

In large heavy saucepan or Dutch oven, heat butter over medium heat; cook celery, onions, garlic, salt and pepper, stirring often, until softened, about 5 minutes.

Add carrots; cook for 4 minutes, stirring occasionally. Add stock and bring to boil; reduce heat, cover and simmer until carrots are tender, about 35 minutes.

In food processor or blender, purée soup, in batches, until smooth. Return to pan and heat through. Stir in dill; ladle into bowls.

SPINACH AND DULSE SOUP

SOUPS AND STEWS › ZUCCHINI, CELERY, SCALLION, DULSE, AVOCADO, SPINACH

SERVES: 4-6

1 zucchini, cut in half-inch cubes

1 stalk celery

1 scallion

1 tablespoon extra virgin olive oil

1/4 cup dulse flakes

1/4 avocado

2 cups spinach leaves, washed

4 cups water

Blend together in a high-speed blender for 3 minutes or until smooth.

Season with sea salt to taste.

Serve with garnish of dulse and a drizzle of olive oil.

SEAFOOD AND BLACK BEAN CHILI

SOUPS AND STEWS › ONION, GREEN&RED PEPPER, POBLANO PEPPER, GARLIC, CHIPOTLE PEPPER, CUMIN, CORIANDER, CHILI POWDER, OREGANO, BLACK BEANS, TOMATO, FISH, SHRIMP, CILANTRO

SERVES: 12

1 teaspoon olive oil

1 onion, finely chopped

1 green pepper, seeded and chopped

1 red pepper, seeded and chopped

1 poblano pepper, seeded and chopped

2 cloves garlic, chopped

1/2 tablespoon sea salt

1/2 teaspoon freshly ground black pepper

2 chipotle peppers in adobo sauce, finely chopped

1 teaspoon ground cumin

1/2 teaspoon ground coriander

1 teaspoon chili powder

1 tablespoon fresh oregano, or 1 teaspoon dried

1 bay leaf

2 x 15-ounces cans black beans, drained and rinsed

3 cups reduced-sodium chicken broth

1 x 28-ounces can no-salt-added diced tomatoes

1 pound mild fish (rock fish, cod or halibut), cut into 1-inch chunks

1/2 pound cooked bay shrimp

Yogurt Cheese to garnish (optional)

fresh cilantro, to garnish

1 lime, cut into wedges

Heat oil in a large soup pot over medium-high heat. Add onion, green, red and poblano peppers, garlic, salt and pepper, and cook until soft, 10 minutes. Add chipotle peppers with sauce, cumin, coriander, chili powder, oregano, bay leaf, beans, broth and tomatoes. Cover and simmer, 20 minutes.

Uncover, remove bay leaf and discard. Increase heat so liquid is briskly simmering. Add fish and gently submerge it into chili using a spoon. Allow fish to cook for three to four minutes until opaque. Taste chili and season with salt and pepper, to taste.

Ladle chili into bowls, top with bay shrimp, Yogurt Cheese and cilantro. Serve with lime wedges to squeeze over top.

TOKYO BEEF AND NOODLE SOUP

SOUPS AND STEWS › SHIITAKE MUSHROOMS, GARLIC, GINGER, LEMONGRASS, CORIANDER, BEEF BROTH, FROZEN VEGETABLES, NOODLES, BEEF SIRLOIN, TOFU, SCALLIONS

SERVES: 4

FOR BROTH:

4 ounces shiitake mushroom stems, rinsed (remove caps and set aside) (can be substituted with dried shiitake mushrooms)

1 tablespoon garlic, minced (about 2–3 cloves)

1 tablespoon ginger, minced

1 stalk lemongrass, crushed (or the zest from 1 lemon: Use a peeler to grate a thin layer of skin off a lemon)

1 tablespoon ground coriander

4 cups low-sodium beef broth

1 tablespoon lite soy sauce

FOR MEAT AND VEGETABLES:

1 bag (12 ounces) frozen vegetable stir-fry

4 ounces shiitake mushrooms caps, rinsed and quartered

8 ounces udon or soba noodles (or substitute angel hair pasta), cooked

1 pound lean beef top sirloin, sliced very thin

4 ounces firm silken tofu, diced

1/4 cup scallions (green onions), rinsed and sliced thin

Thaw frozen vegetables in the microwave (or place entire bag in a bowl of hot water for about 10 minutes). Set aside until step 4.

Combine all ingredients for broth, except soy sauce, in a medium-sized pot or saucepan. Bring to a boil over high heat, then lower heat and simmer for 15 minutes.

Strain the broth through a fine wire colander, and discard the solid parts. Season to taste with soy sauce.

To finish the soup, bring the broth back to a boil. Add the thawed vegetable stir-fry mix and mushroom caps, and simmer for 1 minute.

Add the noodles and continue to simmer for another minute.

Add the beef and continue to simmer for about 5 minutes or until the beef is slightly pink to brown (to a minimum internal temperature of 145 degrees F).

Add tofu and scallions, and simmer 1–2 minutes until heated through.

Serve immediately in 1-cup portions.

SPICED PORK STEW

SOUPS AND STEWS › PICKLING SPICES, BAY LEAF, PORK SHOULDER BUTT, ONION, CELERY, MUSHROOMS, GARLIC, TOMATO PASTE, RED WINE, STEWED TOMATOES, MINT, PARSLEY, MOZZARELLA

SERVES: 6

1 tablespoon pickling spices

1 bay leaf

2 pound pork shoulder butt

1/2 teaspoon each salt and pepper

2 tablespoons vegetable oil

1 onion, sliced

2 stalks celery, chopped

2 cups quartered mushrooms

2 cloves garlic, minced

1/3 cup tomato paste

1 cup dry red wine

1 can (28 ounces) stewed tomatoes

2 tablespoons finely chopped fresh mint

2 tablespoons chopped fresh parsley

1 cup shredded mozzarella cheese

Cut 5-inch (12 cm) double-thickness square of cheesecloth. Place pickling spices and bay leaf in center; tie with string into bundle. Set aside.

Trim and cut pork into 1-inch (2.5 cm) cubes; toss with salt and pepper. In large shallow Dutch oven, heat oil over medium-high heat; brown pork, in batches. Remove to plate.

Drain any fat from pan. Add onion, celery, mushrooms and garlic; fry over medium heat, stirring occasionally, until softened, about 5 minutes. Add tomato paste; cook, stirring, for 2 minutes. Stir in wine, tomatoes and 1/2 cup water, breaking up tomatoes with spoon. Return pork and any accumulated juices to pan. Add spice bundle; bring to boil.

Reduce heat, cover and simmer until pork is tender, about 2 hours. Discard spice bundle.

MOROCCAN CHICKEN STEW WITH COUSCOUS

SOUPS AND STEWS › CHICKEN LEGS, MOROCCAN SPICE, CARROTS, ONION, LEMON JUICE, CHILI, COUSCOUS, MINT

SERVES: 4

1 tablespoon olive oil

1 pound skinless chicken legs, split (about 4 whole legs)

1 tablespoon Moroccan spice blend

1 cup carrots, rinsed, peeled, and diced

1 cup onion, diced

1/4 cup lemon juice

2 cups low-sodium chicken broth

1/2 cup ripe black olives, sliced

1/4 teaspoon salt

1 tablespoon chili sauce (optional)

FOR COUSCOUS:

1 cup low-sodium chicken broth

1 cup couscous (try whole-wheat couscous)

1 tablespoon fresh mint, rinsed, dried, and shredded thin (or 1 teaspoon dried)

Heat olive oil in a large sauté pan. Add chicken legs, and brown on all sides, about 2–3 minutes per side.

Remove chicken from pan and put on a plate with a cover to hold warm.

Add spice blend to sauté pan and toast gently.

Add carrots and onion to sauté pan, and cook for about 3–4 minutes or until the onions have turned clear, but not brown.

Add lemon juice, chicken broth, and olives to sauté pan, and bring to a boil over high heat. Add chicken legs, and return to a boil. Cover and gently simmer for about 10–15 minutes (to a minimum internal temperature of 165 degrees F).

Meanwhile, prepare the couscous by bringing chicken broth to a boil in a saucepan. Add couscous, and remove from the heat. Cover and let stand for 10 minutes.

Fluff couscous with a fork, and gently mix in the mint.

When chicken is cooked, add salt. Serve two chicken legs over ½ cup couscous topped with 1/2 cup sauce in a serving bowl. Add chili sauce to taste.

CHICKEN SOUP

SOUPS AND STEWS › CHICKEN, ONION, CARROTS, CELERY, PARSLEY

SERVES: 6

- one 5-6 pound whole chicken (including giblets)
- 12 cups water
- 4 large yellow onions
- 2 medium carrots
- 2 stalks celery
- 1/4 bunch parsley
- freshly ground black pepper, to taste
- sea salt, to taste

Clean, trim, and quarter the chicken. Peel and chop all the vegetables. Chop parsley leaves.

Place the chicken and giblets in a stockpot, add the water, and bring to a boil. Reduce heat to a simmer and skim off all foam.

Add all the vegetables and parsley, season with salt and pepper, and simmer uncovered for about 3 hours.

Remove the chicken and giblets from the stockpot; discard giblets. Remove the meat from the bones, discard the bones, and return the meat to the soup.

Serve.

QUICK COLD GREEN SOUP

SOUPS AND STEWS › SPINACH, ASPARAGUS, AVOCADO, GREEN ONION, CUCUMBER, LEMON, MINT

SERVES: 4

1/4 pounds spinach, stems removed

1/2 pounds asparagus, cut into 2-inch pieces

1 avocado, chopped

4 green onions, chopped

1 large cucumber, peeled and chopped

2 tablespoons lemon juice

1/4 cup fresh mint leaves

2 cups cold water

freshly ground black pepper, to taste.

Put the asparagus into the blender with 1/2 cup of the water and puree until smooth.

Add the green onions, spinach, cucumber and another 1/2 cup of water. Blend again until smooth.

Add the avocado, lemon juice and mint and repeat blending with the remaining water. Season to taste with pepper. Serve immediately.

CHAPTER 5

Main Dishes

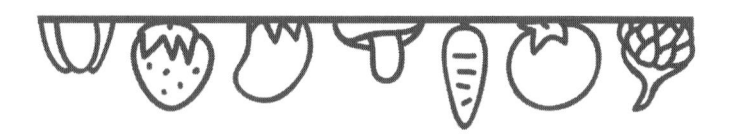

SESAME MAPLE SALMON WITH SPINACH

MAIN DISHES › SALMON FILLETS, MAPLE SYRUP, SPINACH, SCALLION

SERVES: 6

4 teaspoons sesame seeds

6 (6-ounce) salmon fillets

freshly ground black pepper

2 tablespoons pure maple syrup

1/4 cup water

2 bunches spinach

1 scallion, thinly sliced on the bias, for garnish

In a small pan over medium-high heat, toast the sesame seeds while shaking the pan, until they are aromatic and lightly browned. Remove from the heat and set aside.

Preheat the oven to 450 degrees F.

Place the salmon in a large nonstick baking dish. Season lightly with the pepper, then drizzle with the maple syrup.

Bake for 10 to 12 minutes.

While the fish is baking, heat a large skillet over medium-high heat and pour in the water. Add the spinach and cook, tossing, until it is bright green.

Remove the salmon from the oven, sprinkle with the sesame seeds, and serve with the spinach and garnished with scallion.

BRAISED COD WITH LEEKS

MAIN DISHES › CHICKEN, CARROT, CELERY, ROSEMARY, SAGE, BAY

SERVES: 4

1 tablespoon butter

2 cup leeks, split lengthwise, sliced thin, and rinsed well

3 medium carrots, rinsed, peeled, and cut into thin sticks

4 new (red) potatoes, rinsed and sliced into 1/2-inch thick circles

2 cups low-sodium chicken broth

2 tablespoons fresh parsley, rinsed, dried, and chopped (or 2 teaspoons dried)

12 oz cod fillets, cut into 4 portions (3 ounces each)

1/2 teaspoon salt

1/4 teaspoon ground black pepper

Heat butter in a large sauté pan. Add leeks and carrots, and cook gently for 3–5 minutes, stirring often, until the vegetables begin to soften.

Add potatoes, chicken broth, parsley, and salt and pepper, and bring to a boil over high heat. Reduce heat and simmer gently until the vegetables are just tender, about 10–12 minutes.

Add cod fillets, and cover with a tight-fitting lid. Continue cooking over low heat for an additional 5 minutes or until the fish is white and flakes easily with a fork in the thickest part (to a minimum internal temperature of 145 degrees F).

Serve each cod fillet with 1 1/2 cups broth and vegetables.

CLEAN CHICKEN IN A POT

MAIN DISHES › CHICKEN, CARROT, CELERY, ROSEMARY, SAGE, BAY

SERVES: 4

- one whole chicken (2-3 pounds, quartered)
- 2 tablespoons olive oil
- 1 bunch celery
- 4 large carrots
- 4 small spring onions
- 1 fresh rosemary sprig
- 4 fresh sage leaves
- 1 bay leaf
- freshly ground black pepper

Preheat oven to 300 degrees F. Pepper chicken pieces thoroughly and set aside.

Pour olive oil into an oven-proof stockpot and heat over medium flame. Chop carrots, celery, and spring onions into 1-inch pieces. Sauté in olive oil for five minutes.

Add 1 quart of water. Place chicken in the pot. Using kitchen twine, tie together the sage leaves, rosemary, and bay leaf and place in the pot with the chicken. Cover and bake for one hour.

Remove the lid and turn oven setting to broil. Brown chicken for 5 minutes. Remove from oven and serve with broth and vegetables.

GRILLED CHICKEN BREASTS WITH GARLIC

MAIN DISHES › CHICKEN BREAST, GARLIC, LEMON, VINEGAR

SERVES: 4

4 boneless, skinless organic chicken breast chicken breasts
3 garlic cloves
1 cup olive or coconut oil
juice from 1 lemon
1 cup apple cider vinegar

Crush and mince the garlic cloves.

Combine the olive oil, lemon juice and vinegar together in a gallon-sized Ziploc bag.

Put the chicken breasts into the bag and seal.

Marinate in the refrigerator for 3 hours.

Preheat your grill to medium heat about 10 - 15 minutes before time to grill.

Gently shake off the marinade from the chicken and place onto heated grill.

Grill until fully cooked.

GRILLED SCALLOPS WITH SAUTÉED ASPARAGUS AND PEPPERS

MAIN DISHES › SCALLOPS, RED PEPPER, BABY ASPARAGUS, CUMIN, PAPRIKA, TURMERIC, ONION POWDER

SERVES: 4

1 pound wild caught large scallops

1/8 teaspoon sea salt

1/8 teaspoon freshly ground black pepper

1 teaspoon olive oil

1 red pepper, seeded and thinly sliced

1 yellow or orange pepper, seeded and thinly sliced

2 cups baby asparagus, sliced into 3-inch-long pieces (match length of sliced peppers)

1/4 teaspoon ground cumin

1/4 teaspoon paprika

1/4 teaspoon turmeric

1/4 teaspoon onion powder

Heat a large cast iron skillet over high heat. Make sure scallops are dry then season with a pinch of salt and pepper. Add scallops to dry skillet, turn heat down to medium and cook two minutes on each side until slightly charred and tender. Remove and set aside.

Return skillet to stove and add olive oil. Add peppers, asparagus, cumin, paprika, turmeric and onion powder. Season with a pinch of salt and pepper, and sauté until tender-crisp, three minutes.

Divide vegetables equally among four plates and top with scallops.

THYME ROASTED TURKEY BREASTS

MAIN DISHES › TURKEY BREAST, ONION, THYME, CELERY, PARSLEY

SERVES: 10

1 (6-7-pound) turkey breast, skin on

2 large onions, thinly sliced

1/2 tablespoon freshly ground black pepper

1/2 cup minced thyme

1/2 tablespoon celery flakes

1/2 tablespoon dried parsley

1/2 tablespoon mustard seed

Arrange the onion slices in a thin layer on the bottom of a 6- or 7-quart slow cooker.

Make a small slit in the skin of the turkey and spread the thyme between the skin and meat. Smooth the skin back onto the turkey.

In a small bowl, stir the pepper, parsley, celery flakes, and mustard seed. Rub the spice mixture onto the skin of the turkey.

Place the turkey in the slow cooker on top of the onion layer. Cook for 8 hours. Remove the skin and onions and discard them before serving the turkey.

MARINATED FLANK STEAK

MAIN DISHES › FLANK STEAK, GINGER, ORANGE JUICE, SESAME OIL

SERVES: 4

1 pound flank steak (preferably organic)

1 1/2 cups freshly squeezed orange juice

1 tablespoon toasted sesame oil

1/4 cup ume plum vinegar

1 tablespoon peeled and minced fresh ginger

1 teaspoon minced fresh garlic

In a small bowl, combine the orange juice, vinegar, sesame oil, ginger, and garlic to make the marinade. Pour the marinade into an 11 by 7-inch baking dish, then place the flank steak in the dish. Marinate for 4 to 8 hours in the refrigerator, turning it halfway through the marinating time if desired.

Remove the steak from the refrigerator and let rest for 15 minutes. Heat a large skillet over high heat. Cook the steak for 2 to 4 minutes on each side until an instant-read thermometer inserted into the thickest part of the steak registers 130 degrees F for medium-rare, or until cooked to your desired doneness.

Let the steak rest for 5 to 10 minutes. Cut against the grain into 1/2-inch-thick slices and serve.

LETTUCE-WRAPPED BEEF AND PEPPER FAJITAS

MAIN DISHES › SIRLOIN STEAK, CHILI, RED&GREEN PEPPER, ONION, SALSA, LIME JUICE, LETTUCE

SERVES: 4

1 pound top sirloin grilling steak

1 teaspoon chili powder

1/2 teaspoon salt

1 teaspoon vegetable oil

1 each sweet red and green pepper, thinly sliced

1 onion, sliced

2 cloves garlic, minced

1/2 cup salsa

1 tablespoon lime or lemon juice

1/4 cup light sour cream

8 lettuce leaves

Trim fat off steak; sprinkle with half each of the chili powder and salt. Broil steak, turning once, until browned but still pink inside, about 6 minutes. Transfer to cutting board and tent with foil; let stand for 10 minutes before slicing thinly across the grain.

Meanwhile, brush vegetable oil over nonstick skillet over medium heat; cook red and green peppers, sliced onion, minced garlic and remaining chili powder and salt, stirring occasionally, until tender-crisp, about 4 minutes. Stir in salsa and lime juice.

Mound vegetables, steak and sour cream in each lettuce leaf; roll up.

PORK MEDALLIONS AND PEPPERS

MAIN DISHES › PORK TENDERLOIN, GARLIC, YELLOW/RED BELL PEPPER, LIME JUICE, ROSEMARY

SERVES: 4

1 pound pork tenderloin, cut into 1-inch medallions

2 cloves garlic, peeled and minced

1/2 teaspoon sea salt

1/2 teaspoon freshly ground black pepper

1 tablespoon olive oil

1 large yellow bell pepper, seeded, deribbed and sliced

1 large red bell pepper, seeded, deribbed and sliced

1 teaspoon lime juice

1 teaspoon finely minced fresh rosemary, plus 1 teaspoon for garnishing

2 teaspoons balsamic vinegar

Sprinkle the salt and pepper on the pork medallions.

In a large skillet that is already hot, heat the oil over medium-high heat and add the pork. Cook for 5 minutes and then flip.

Reduce the heat to medium, add the peppers, garlic and 1 teaspoon of the rosemary, and cook for another 8 minutes, or until the pork is cooked through.

Combine the lime juice and vinegar in a small bowl and pour over the pork. Top with the remaining 1 teaspoon rosemary.

LEG OF LAMB

MAIN DISHES › LEG OF LAMB, GARLIC, ROSEMARY, RED WINE

SERVES: 6

- 1 (4-pound) bone-in leg of lamb
- 2 tablespoons olive oil
- 5 cloves garlic, cut into spears
- 1/2 teaspoon ground pepper
- 1 tablespoon dried rosemary
- 4 cups chicken broth
- 1/4 cup dry red wine

Make small incisions evenly over the lamb. Place garlic spears into the incisions in the lamb.

Rub olive oil, rosemary, and pepper over the lamb. Place lamb into a greased 4- or 6-quart slow cooker.

Pour broth and wine around the leg of lamb. Cook on high for 4 hours or on low for 8 hours.

Serve the roast lamb in bowls. Ladle the sauce from the slow cooker over each serving.

GRILLED LAMB CHOPS

MAIN DISHES › LAMB CHOPS, LEMON, GARLIC, OREGANO

SERVES: 3

6 organic lamb chops

3 cloves garlic, minced

1/4 cup olive oil

2 tablespoons lemon juice

1 teaspoon dried oregano

1 small shallot, minced

freshly ground black pepper, to taste

In a small bowl, combine the olive oil, lemon juice, garlic, shallot and oregano. Season with freshly ground black pepper to taste. Stir to combine well.

Put the lamb chops and the marinade in a gallon freezer bag and shake. Chill for at least 1 hour, and up to 24.

When ready to cook, preheat grill to high heat. Grill the chops for about 5 minutes per side. Allow to rest for 10 minutes and serve.

Place mushrooms in the slow cooker. Cover. Cook on High for 2 hours.

CHAPTER 6

Vegetables

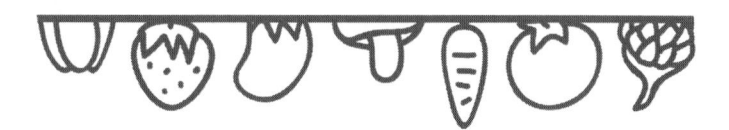

BRUSSELS SPROUTS WITH LEMON

VEGETABLES › BRUSSELS SPROUTS, LEMON JUICE, LEMON ZEST

SERVES: 4

1/2 cup water

5 cups quartered Brussels sprouts

sea salt and freshly ground black pepper

1 tablespoon extra-virgin olive oil

1 tablespoon freshly squeezed lemon juice

1 teaspoon lemon zest

Put the water and Brussels sprouts in a large skillet over medium heat. Bring to a simmer and cover the skillet.

Cook until the Brussels sprouts are tender but still crisp, 5 to 8 minutes. Most of the water should be evaporated. Season with a pinch of the salt and pepper.

Increase the heat to medium-high and add the oil to the skillet.

Cook without stirring for about 5 minutes, until the Brussels sprouts are lightly caramelized on the underside.

Remove the skillet from the heat and stir in the lemon juice and zest. Serve alongside chicken or beef.

VEGGIE MEDLEY

VEGETABLES › CAULIFLOWER, BROCCOLI, BABY CARROTS, ONION, GARLIC, OREGANO

SERVES: 4

4 garlic cloves, finely chopped

1/2 sweet onion, thinly sliced

1 teaspoon dried tarragon

4 tablespoons extra virgin olive oil

1 teaspoon dried oregano

1 cup cauliflower florets

1 cup broccoli florets

1 cup diced baby carrots

lemon wedges, to taste

freshly ground pepper, to taste

Heat olive oil in a cast iron skillet over medium flame. Add onion, garlic, tarragon, and oregano and sauté while stirring for two to three minutes. Add broccoli, cauliflower, and carrots and continue cooking for three to four minutes.

Once the veggies begin to stick to the pan, stir and continue cooking until slightly charred. Turn off heat and cover; let sit for five minutes.

Squeeze lemon wedges over veggies, drizzling juice evenly. Sprinkle with freshly ground pepper.

SAUTEED SPINACH

VEGETABLES › SPINACH, GARLIC, NUTMEG, EXTRA-VIRGIN OLIVE OIL

SERVES: 4

- **1 tablespoon extra-virgin olive oil**
- **4 teaspoons minced garlic**
- **8 cups fresh spinach**
- **1/4 teaspoon nutmeg**

Place a large skillet over medium-high heat and add the olive oil.

Saute the garlic until it's fragrant, about 2 minutes.

Add the spinach and cook until it's wilted, about 2 minutes.

Season with the nutmeg and serve alongside your favorite protein.

PARMESAN ASPARAGUS

VEGETABLES › ASPARAGUS, PARMESAN, BREAD CRUMBS

SERVES: 4

1 pound asparagus, trimmed

2 tablespoons grated Parmesan cheese

2 tablespoons toasted bread crumbs

1 tablespoon extra-virgin olive oil

1/4 teaspoon each salt and pepper

In large pot of boiling salted water, cook asparagus until tender, about 5 minutes. Drain and toss with cheese, bread crumbs, oil, salt and pepper.

BALSAMIC ROSEMARY BEETS

VEGETABLES › BEETS, BALSAMIC VINEGAR, ROSEMARY

SERVES: 4

4 medium beets, peeled and cut into 1-inch cubes (about 4 cups)

1 tablespoon balsamic vinegar

1 tablespoon olive oil

1/2 teaspoon freshly ground black pepper

1 tablespoon minced fresh rosemary

1/4 teaspoon sea salt

Preheat the oven to 400 degrees F.

In a medium bowl, combine the beets, olive oil, vinegar, rosemary, pepper, and salt. Transfer the beets to a 9 by 13-inch baking dish and cover with aluminum foil.

Bake for 45 minutes. Remove the foil and bake, uncovered, for 10 to 20 more minutes, until the beets are tender when pierced with a fork, then serve.

BAKED TOMATOES GRATIN

VEGETABLES › PLUM TOMATOES, BREAD CRUMBS, GARLIC, ITALIAN PARSLEY

SERVES: 4

6 large plum tomatoes (about 1 1/2 pound total)

1/4 cup extra-virgin olive oil

1/2 teaspoon each salt and pepper

2 cups fresh bread crumbs

2 cloves garlic, minced

1/4 cup chopped fresh Italian parsley

Cut each tomato lengthwise into 6 wedges. In bowl, toss tomato wedges with half each of the oil, salt and pepper.

Arrange tomatoes, cut side up, in 13- x 9-inch (3 L) glass baking dish; roast in 400 degrees F oven for 30 minutes.

Meanwhile, in bowl, combine bread crumbs, garlic, parsley and remaining oil, salt and pepper.

Remove tomatoes from oven; sprinkle with bread-crumb mixture. Roast until bread-crumb mixture is golden, about 20 minutes.

CHAPTER 7

Desserts

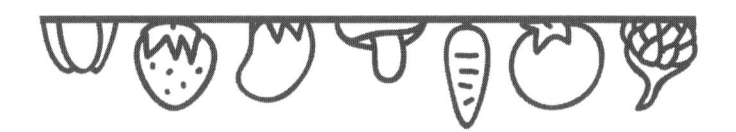

MELON COOLER

DESSERTS › HONEYDEW MELON, LIME, HONEY, COCONUT WATER, MINT, ICE

SERVES: 4

- 2 cups honeydew melon cubes
- 1 cup coconut water
- 1/2 cup lime juice
- 1/2 cup ice cubes
- 1 teaspoon honey
- 1/4 cup fresh mint leaves

Puree the melon cubes and the lime juice in a blender until smooth.

Add the remaining ingredients and puree again.

GRILLED PINEAPPLE WITH CIN-NAMON YOGURT SAUCE

DESSERTS › PINEAPPLE, CINNAMON, HONEY, GREEK YOGURT

SERVES: 6

extra-virgin olive oil for the grill

1 cup nonfat plain Greek yogurt

2 tablespoons honey

1 teaspoon ground cinnamon

1 pineapple, skinned, cored, and sliced into 1-inch slices

Preheat the grill to medium heat.

Lightly oil the grill.

In a small bowl, stir together the yogurt, honey, and cinnamon; set aside.

Lay the pineapple slices on the grill and cook for 3 minutes.

Flip the pineapple over and grill for another 3 minutes.

Arrange the pineapple on 6 plates and serve drizzled with the honey yogurt.

CHERRY BERRY

DESSERTS › CHERRIES, RASPBERRIES, BLUEBERRIES, BLACKBERRIES, VANILLA, CLOVE, CINNAMON, MINT

SERVES: 4

1/2 cup Bing or Rainier cherries, pitted and chopped
1/2 cup golden raspberries
1/2 cup blueberries
1/2 cup blackberries
1 teaspoon vanilla extract
1/2 teaspoon clove powder
1/2 teaspoon ground cinnamon
1 tablespoon chopped fresh mint leaves, plus 4 leaves for garnish

Combine cherries and berries in a medium bowl. Add vanilla, clove, cinnamon, and chopped mint and gently toss. Chill for thirty minutes. Garnish with mint leaves just before serving.

STRAWBERRY PEACH PARFAITS

DESSERTS › VANILLA YOGURT, STRAWBERRIES, PEACHES, CINNAMON

SERVES: 4

4 cups frozen vanilla yogurt

4 whole strawberries

STRAWBERRY PEACH SAUCE:

2 cups sliced peeled peaches or nectarines

1/4 cup brown sugar

pinch cinnamon

1 cup sliced strawberries

STRAWBERRY PEACH SAUCE: In saucepan, bring peaches, sugar and cinnamon to boil over medium heat. Reduce heat and simmer, stirring gently once or twice, until peaches are tender, about 10 minutes. Add sliced strawberries; let cool.

In 4 parfait glasses or bowls, alternately layer sauce with frozen yogurt. Garnish with whole strawberries.

BANANA COCONUT ICE CREAM

DESSERTS › BANANA, COCONUT, COCONUT MILK

SERVES: 6

6 bananas

1 (13.5-ounce) can light coconut milk

3/4 cup unsweetened shredded coconut

Peel and slice the bananas.

Put the banana chunks in a large container and freeze overnight.

Transfer the frozen banana to a food processor or blender and process with the coconut milk until smooth and creamy.

Serve immediately, topped with the shredded coconut.

PUMPKIN PIE PUDDINGS

DESSERTS › PUMPKIN, HONEY, EGG WHITE, CINNAMON, GINGER, CLOVES, ALMOND MILK

SERVES: 6

1 cup canned pumpkin (not pumpkin pie mix)
2 tablespoons honey
2 egg whites, lightly beaten
1/2 teaspoon ground cinnamon
1/4 teaspoon ground ginger
1/8 teaspoon ground cloves
1 cup unsweetened almond milk

Preheat the oven to 425 degrees F.

Put six 4-ounce ramekins in a baking dish.

Combine all the ingredients in a large mixing bowl and whisk to blend well.

Pour the mixture evenly into the ramekins.

Add water to the baking dish to reach about 1 inch up the sides of the ramekins, taking care not to get any water in the batter.

Bake for 15 minutes, then reduce the heat to 350 degrees F.

Bake for 30 to 35 more minutes, until the puddings are set.

Remove from the oven and cool completely.

CHAPTER 8

Smoothies

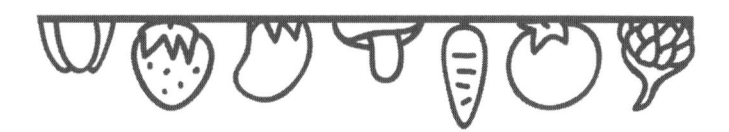

CLEAN BREEZE SMOOTHIE

SMOOTHIES › CUCUMBER, KIWI, KOMBUCHA, GREEK YOGURT, CILANTRO

SERVES: 2

1 small cucumber, chopped

2 ripe kiwis, peeled

1 cup ginger-flavored kombucha

1/2 cup low-fat plain Greek yogurt

2 tablespoons fresh cilantro leaves

6 ice cubes

Combine cucumber, kiwis, kombucha, yogurt, cilantro and ice cubes in blender; blend until smooth. Serve immediately.

NUTTY BERRY SMOOTHIE

SMOOTHIES › STRAWBERRIES, CASHEWS, SUNFLOWER SEEDS, HEMP SEEDS, ALMOND MILK

SERVES: 2

2 cups sliced strawberries

2 tablespoons chopped cashews

1 tablespoon sunflower seeds

1 tablespoon hemp seeds

1 cup vanilla almond milk

In a blender, process all the ingredients until smooth. Serve in a tall glass.

MANGO-KALE STARTER

SMOOTHIES › BABY SPINACH, KALE, MANGO, COCONUT WATER

SERVES: 1

3 cups baby spinach
1 cup kale
1/2 ripe mango, pitted, sliced
1 cup coconut water

Add the spinach, kale, and ripe mango. Juice, then add the coconut water, whisking well to combine.

BANANA SPICE SMOOTHIE

SMOOTHIES › BANANA, KEFIR, CINNAMON, NUTMEG, ALLSPICE

SERVES: 2

2 ripe bananas
2 cups vanilla kefir
1/2 teaspoon ground cinnamon
1/8 teaspoon ground nutmeg
1/8 teaspoon ground allspice
12 ice cubes

Combine kefir, bananas, cinnamon, nutmeg, allspice and ice cubes in a blender; blend until smooth. Serve immediately.

PEAR GREEN TEA SMOOTHIE

SMOOTHIES › BABY SPINACH, KALE, MANGO, COCONUT WATER

SERVES: 2

- 2 pears, cored and chopped
- 2 cups coconut milk
- 2 tablespoons green tea powder, stirred into 2 tablespoons hot water
- 1 1/2 cups ice cubes

In a blender, process all the ingredients until smooth. Serve in a tall glass.

GREEN APPLE SMOOTHIE

SMOOTHIES › KALE, BABY SPINACH, APPLE

SERVES: 4

1 cup coconut water

1 cup kale

1 cup baby spinach

1 1/2 Fuji apples, cored

1/8 teaspoon cinnamon

1/8 teaspoon nutmeg

1 cup ice

dash of flaxseed or chia seeds (optional)

Add ingredients into a blender and blend until smooth.

GINGER PINEAPPLE GREEN

SMOOTHIES › PINEAPPLE, BABY SPINACH, GINGER, CUCUMBER

SERVES: 2

- 3/4 cup fresh pineapple
- 3 cups baby spinach
- 1 tablespoon fresh ginger
- 1 medium cucumber

Add all ingredients into a juicer and juice. Then whisk in cinnamon.

GREEN SMOOTHIE

SMOOTHIES › BANANA, PEAR/APPLE, KALE, ORANGE JUICE, COLD WATER, FLAXSEED

SERVES: 2

2 ripe medium bananas

1 ripe pear or apple, peeled if desired, chopped

2 cups chopped kale leaves, tough stems removed

1/2 cup cold orange juice

1/2 cup cold water

1 tablespoon ground flaxseed

12 ice cubes

Place bananas, pear (or apple), kale, orange juice, water, ice cubes and flaxseed in a blender. Pulse a few times, then puree until smooth, scraping down the sides as necessary.

STANDARD U.S./METRIC MEASUREMENT CONVERSIONS

VOLUME CONVERSIONS U.S. Volume	Metric Equivalent
1/8 teaspoon	0.5 milliliter
1/4 teaspoon	1 milliliter
1/2 teaspoon	2 milliliters
1 teaspoon	5 milliliters
1/2 tablespoon	7 milliliters
1 tablespoon (3 teaspoons)	15 milliliters
2 tablespoons (1 fluid ounce)	30 milliliters
1/4 cup (4 tablespoons)	60 milliliters
1/3 cup	90 milliliters
1/2 cup (4 fluid ounces)	125 milliliters
2/3 cup	160 milliliters
3/4 cup (6 fluid ounces)	180 milliliters

VOLUME CONVERSIONS

U.S. Volume	Metric Equivalent
1 cup (16 tablespoons)	250 milliliters
1 pint (2 cups)	500 milliliters
1 quart (4 cups)	1 liter (about)

WEIGHT CONVERSIONS

U.S. Weight	Metric Equivalent
1/2 ounce	15 grams
1 ounce	30 grams
2 ounces	60 grams
3 ounces	85 grams
1/4 pound (4 ounces)	115 grams
1/2 pound (8 ounces)	225 grams
3/4 pound (12 ounces)	340 grams
1 pound (16 ounces)	454 grams

Desserts

OVEN TEMPERATURE CONVERSIONS

Degrees Fahrenheit	Degrees Celsius
200 degrees F	95 degrees C
250 degrees F	120 degrees C
275 degrees F	135 degrees C
300 degrees F	150 degrees C
325 degrees F	160 degrees C
350 degrees F	180 degrees C
375 degrees F	190 degrees C
400 degrees F	205 degrees C
425 degrees F	220 degrees C
450 degrees F	230 degrees C